DR. STEPHANIE D. WARD

Preventing Suicide in Your Loved Ones

How to Spot the Signs and Help Them Get the Help They Need

Contents

About the Author

Dr. Stephanie D. Ward is a compassionate and dedicated mental health professional who has devoted her career to helping individuals who have struggled with suicide. With her extensive knowledge, expertise, and unwavering commitment to making a difference, Dr. Ward has become a beacon of hope for those in need.

Dr. Ward holds a Ph.D. in Clinical Psychology and has specialized in the field of suicide prevention and intervention for over a decade. Her passion for this work stems from a deep understanding of the profound impact that suicide can have on individuals, families, and communities.

Throughout her career, Dr. Ward has worked tirelessly to provide support, guidance, and healing to those who have faced the darkest moments of their lives. She has helped countless individuals find their strength, rediscover hope, and navigate the complexities of mental health challenges. Her empathetic and non-judgmental approach creates a safe space for her clients to share their deepest fears and vulnerabilities.

As an author, Dr. Ward strives to share her knowledge and insights with a wider audience. Through her writing, she aims to increase awareness, reduce stigma, and provide practical guidance for those who may be struggling or supporting someone in need. Her hope is that this book will serve as a valuable resource, offering a compassionate and informed perspective on recognizing the warning signs of suicide.

Introduction

In the depths of despair, when darkness seems to engulf our loved ones, it is our duty to be their guiding light. Suicide, a haunting reality that affects far too many lives, demands our attention and action. It is a topic that often shrouds itself in silence, leaving families and communities grappling with the devastating aftermath. But it doesn't have to be this way. We have the power to make a difference, to prevent the unimaginable, and to save lives.

As I sit here, pen in hand, pouring my heart onto these pages, I am driven by a deeply personal motivation to address the urgent need for suicide prevention. You see, I have witnessed the pain and despair that suicide leaves in its wake. I have felt the weight of loss, the ache of unanswered questions, and the relentless torment of wondering if there was something more I could have done. It is this profound experience that has ignited a fire within me to share knowledge, compassion, and hope.

This book, "Preventing Suicide in Your Loved Ones: How to Spot the Signs and Help Them Get the Help They Need," is not just a compilation of facts and strategies. It is a testament to the power of love, understanding, and intervention. It is a call to action for each and every one of us to become agents of change, to be vigilant in recognizing the signs, and to extend a lifeline to those teetering on the edge.

Suicide prevention is not a solitary endeavor; it requires a collective effort. Together, we can create a world where no one feels alone, where mental health is prioritized, and where lives are saved. Through education, awareness, and unwavering support, we can dismantle the stigma that surrounds suicide and create a society that nurtures resilience, fosters hope, and celebrates life.

In the pages that follow, we will embark on a journey of understanding, compassion, and empowerment. We will explore the warning signs, learn how to have difficult conversations, and discover the resources available to help those in need. We will delve into the importance of mental health and self-care, and explore strategies to build resilience in individuals and communities. We will challenge the stigma, advocate for change, and share inspiring stories of hope and recovery.

My hope is that this book will serve as a guiding light for you, equipping you with the knowledge, tools, and confidence to make a difference in the lives of your loved ones. Together, let us embark on this mission of prevention, armed with compassion, understanding, and a determination to save lives.

Understanding Suicide

Suicide. A word that carries immense weight and evokes a myriad of emotions. It is an act that defies comprehension, leaving in its wake a trail of heartbreak and unanswered questions. But what exactly is suicide, and how does it impact individuals and communities?

At its core, suicide is the tragic and deliberate act of ending one's own life. It is a desperate attempt to escape unbearable pain, anguish, or a sense of hopelessness. The impact of suicide is far-reaching, extending beyond the individual who is lost. It ripples through families, friends, and entire communities, leaving a profound void that can never be filled.

Statistics and prevalence of suicide

To truly understand the gravity of the issue, we must confront the stark reality of suicide's prevalence. The numbers paint a sobering picture, revealing the urgent need for action and prevention. According to the World Health Organization (WHO), approximately 800,000 people die by suicide each year, making it a leading cause of death worldwide. That means, on average, one person dies by suicide every 40 seconds.

These statistics are not mere numbers; they represent lives cut short, dreams extinguished, and potential unrealized. They remind us of the urgency to address this silent epidemic and to create a world where lives are cherished and preserved.

<u>The connection between mental health and suicide</u>

While suicide is a complex issue with multifaceted causes, there is a strong and undeniable link between mental health and suicide. Mental health struggles, such as depression, anxiety, bipolar disorder, and substance abuse, can significantly increase the risk of suicidal thoughts and behaviors.

Imagine a person trapped in the depths of depression, feeling as though they are drowning in a sea of darkness. The weight of their pain becomes unbearable, and suicide may seem like the only escape. It is crucial to recognize that mental health conditions are not character flaws or signs of weakness; they are legitimate medical conditions that require understanding, support, and treatment.

By acknowledging the connection between mental health and suicide, we can begin to dismantle the stigma surrounding mental illness. We can foster a society that prioritizes mental well-being, offers accessible resources, and promotes early intervention. It is through this collective effort that we can save lives and provide hope to those who need it most.

Understanding suicide is not an easy task. It requires us to confront uncomfortable truths and challenge societal norms. But by delving into the depths of this complex issue, we equip ourselves with the knowledge and empathy needed to make a difference. Together, let us strive for a world where suicide is prevented, lives are saved, and every individual feels valued, supported, and understood.

Recognizing the Warning Signs

When it comes to suicide prevention, one of the most crucial steps is being able to recognize the warning signs. By understanding and identifying these signs, we can intervene and provide the support and help that individuals in distress desperately need. While it's important to remember that every person is unique and may exhibit different signs, there are some common warning signs to be aware of:

Changes in behavior: Pay attention to significant changes in behavior, such as withdrawal from social activities, increased isolation, or a sudden loss of interest in hobbies or passions.

Extreme mood swings: Noticeable shifts in mood, from extreme sadness and despair to sudden bursts of anger or irritability, can be indicative of emotional distress.

Talking about death or suicide: Take any mention of death or suicide seriously. Statements like "I wish I wasn't here anymore" or "Everyone would be better off without me" should never be ignored.

Giving away belongings: If someone starts giving away their

prized possessions or making arrangements as if they won't be around, it could be a sign that they are contemplating suicide.

Increased substance abuse: Escalating or excessive use of drugs or alcohol can be a way for individuals to cope with their emotional pain.

Behavioral, emotional, and verbal cues to watch for

In addition to the common warning signs, it's important to be attentive to specific behavioral, emotional, and verbal cues that may indicate someone is at risk for suicide. These cues can manifest in various ways and may include:

Expressing feelings of hopelessness: Listen for statements that convey a sense of hopelessness, such as "There's no way out" or "I can't go on like this."

Withdrawing from loved ones: Notice if someone starts isolating themselves from family and friends, avoiding social interactions, or becoming increasingly distant.

Sudden calmness: Sometimes, individuals who have been struggling with intense emotional pain may exhibit a sudden calmness or a sense of peace. This can be a sign that they have made a decision to end their life.

Engaging in risky behaviors: Reckless actions, such as driving recklessly, participating in dangerous activities without concern for personal safety, or engaging in self-harm, can be red flags.

Drastic changes in appearance: Pay attention to significant changes in appearance, hygiene, or self-care. Neglecting personal grooming or a sudden disinterest in appearance may indicate emotional distress.

The role of risk factors and protective factors

Understanding the role of risk factors and protective factors is essential in recognizing the warning signs of suicide. Risk factors are conditions or circumstances that increase an individual's vulnerability to suicidal thoughts and behaviors. Some common risk factors include:

Mental health disorders: Conditions like depression, anxiety, bipolar disorder, schizophrenia, and substance abuse significantly increase the risk of suicide.

Previous suicide attempts: Individuals who have previously attempted suicide are at a higher risk of future attempts.

Family history of suicide: Having a family member who has died by suicide increases the likelihood of suicidal ideation and attempts.

Access to lethal means: Easy access to firearms, medications, or other lethal methods can increase the risk of completed suicide.

On the other hand, protective factors are elements that can help mitigate the risk of suicide. These include:

Strong social support: Having a network of supportive relationships, such as family, friends, or community connections, can provide a buffer against suicidal thoughts.

Access to mental health care: Timely access to mental health services and effective treatment options can be crucial in preventing suicide.

Problem-solving skills: Individuals who possess strong problem-solving skills and coping mechanisms are better equipped to navigate challenging situations.

Positive connections to community and culture: Feeling a sense of belonging and connection to one's community or cultural identity can provide a protective factor against suicide.

By understanding these warning signs, behavioral cues, and the interplay of risk and protective factors, we can become more adept at recognizing when someone may be in crisis. Remember, it's important to approach these situations with empathy, compassion, and a willingness to listen. If you suspect someone may be at risk for suicide, don't hesitate to reach out, offer support, and help them access the appropriate resources. Together, we can make a difference and save lives.

Having Difficult Conversations

In the realm of suicide prevention, having difficult conversations is not only important but essential. It is through open and honest communication that we can break down barriers, offer support, and potentially save lives. However, these conversations can be challenging, uncomfortable, and emotionally charged. Yet, it is precisely in these moments of discomfort that we have the opportunity to make a profound impact.

Open and honest communication creates a safe space for individuals to express their thoughts, fears, and struggles without judgment. It allows us to gain insight into their experiences and emotions, enabling us to provide the support they need. By fostering an environment of trust and understanding, we can encourage those who are struggling to share their pain and seek help.

Strategies for initiating conversations about suicide

Initiating conversations about suicide requires sensitivity, empathy, and careful consideration of the individual's well-being. Here are some strategies to help navigate these difficult discussions:

Choose the right time and place: Find a quiet and private setting where the person feels comfortable and safe. Ensure that you have enough time for an uninterrupted conversation.

Express concern and empathy: Begin the conversation by expressing genuine concern for the person's well-being. Let them know that you care and are there to listen without judgment.

Use open-ended questions: Encourage the person to share their thoughts and feelings by asking open-ended questions. This allows them to express themselves freely and provides you with a deeper understanding of their experiences.

Listen actively: Practice active listening by giving your full attention to the person speaking. Maintain eye contact, nod to show understanding, and avoid interrupting. Reflect back their feelings and thoughts to demonstrate that you are truly listening.

Avoid judgment and criticism: It is crucial to create a non-judgmental and safe space for the person to open up. Avoid making negative comments or expressing criticism, as this can further isolate them.

Offer support and resources: Let the person know that they are not alone and that help is available. Provide information about mental health resources, helplines, or professional support services that they can turn to.

<u>Active listening and empathy</u>

Active listening and empathy are vital components of having difficult conversations about suicide. They allow us to truly connect with the person in distress and provide the support they need. Here's how you can practice active listening and empathy:

Be present: Give your undivided attention to the person speaking. Put aside distractions and focus solely on them.

Validate their feelings: Acknowledge and validate the person's emotions. Let them know that their feelings are valid and understandable.

Reflect and paraphrase: Repeat or paraphrase what the person has said to ensure that you understand their perspective correctly. This shows that you are actively engaged in the conversation.

Avoid offering solutions: Instead of jumping to provide solutions, focus on listening and understanding. Sometimes, individuals simply need a compassionate ear to share their burden.

Show empathy: Put yourself in the person's shoes and try to understand their experience from their point of view. Offer words of empathy and reassurance to let them know they are not alone.

Having difficult conversations about suicide is not about fixing someone's problems or providing all the answers. It is about creating a space for open dialogue, active listening, and empathy. By approaching these conversations with care and compassion, we can offer support, help individuals feel heard, and guide them towards the resources they need to find hope and healing.

Assessing Risk and Seeking Help

When faced with a situation where someone may be at risk for suicide, it is crucial to conduct a thorough risk assessment. Assessing the level of risk helps us determine the appropriate course of action and ensure the person's safety. Here are some key steps to consider when conducting a suicide risk assessment:

Establish rapport: Build trust and create a safe space for open communication. Let the person know that you are there to support them without judgment.

Ask direct questions: While it may feel uncomfortable, it is important to ask direct questions about suicide. Ask if they are having thoughts of suicide, if they have a plan, and if they have access to the means to carry it out.

Assess the severity of risk: Evaluate the severity of risk by considering factors such as the presence of a plan, access to lethal means, previous suicide attempts, and the level of distress the person is experiencing.

Identify protective factors: Look for protective factors that can mitigate the risk of suicide. These may include a strong support system, access to mental health resources, problem-solving skills, and a sense of purpose.

Involve professionals: If the risk is high or imminent, involve mental health professionals, such as therapists, counselors, or crisis hotlines, who are trained to handle these situations.

Identifying appropriate resources and support systems

Identifying appropriate resources and support systems is a crucial step in helping individuals at risk for suicide. Here are some key resources and support systems to consider:

Crisis hotlines: Provide the person with the contact information for local or national crisis hotlines. These helplines are staffed by trained professionals who can offer immediate support and guidance.

Mental health professionals: Encourage the person to seek help from mental health professionals, such as therapists, counselors, or psychiatrists. These professionals can provide ongoing support and treatment.

Support groups: Connect the person with support groups or peer networks where they can find understanding, empathy, and shared experiences. Support groups can offer a sense of community and validation.

Community resources: Research and provide information about local community resources, such as mental health clinics, nonprofit organizations, or faith-based organizations that offer counseling or support services.

Emergency services: In cases of immediate danger, do not hesitate to call emergency services. They are trained to handle crisis situations and can provide the necessary intervention and support.

<u>Encouraging professional help-seeking</u>

Encouraging individuals at risk for suicide to seek professional help is crucial for their well-being and safety. Here are some strategies to encourage professional help-seeking:

Normalize seeking help: Emphasize that seeking help is a sign of strength, not weakness. Let the person know that many people face challenges and that reaching out for support is a courageous step.

Share success stories: Share stories of individuals who have sought professional help and experienced positive outcomes. Hearing about others' journeys can inspire hope and reduce stigma.

Offer assistance: Offer to help the person find a mental health professional, make appointments, or accompany them to their first session. Assure them that they don't have to navigate the process alone.

Highlight the benefits: Discuss the potential benefits of professional help, such as gaining coping strategies, developing a safety plan, and receiving evidence-based treatment options tailored to their needs.

Reinforce ongoing support: Remind the person that seeking professional help is not a one-time fix. Encourage them to engage in ongoing therapy or counseling to address underlying issues and build resilience.

Providing Immediate Support

When faced with a crisis situation involving someone at risk for suicide, it is crucial to respond promptly and effectively. Here are some key steps to consider when providing immediate support:

Stay calm and present: It's important to remain calm and composed, even in the face of a crisis. This will help create a sense of stability and reassurance for the person in distress.

Listen actively: Give the person your full attention and actively listen to their concerns. Allow them to express their emotions and thoughts without interruption or judgment.

Validate their feelings: Validate the person's feelings and let them know that it's okay to feel the way they do. Show empathy and understanding, reassuring them that they are not alone.

Ask about their safety: Inquire about their immediate safety. If they have a plan or access to lethal means, take it seriously and ensure their safety by removing any potential harm.

Avoid leaving them alone: If the person is in immediate danger or at high risk, do not leave them alone. Stay with them or ensure that someone trustworthy and supportive is present.

<u>Safety planning and creating a supportive environment</u>

Creating a supportive environment and developing a safety plan can help individuals at risk for suicide feel more secure and provide them with a sense of control. Here are some strategies to consider:

Collaborate on a safety plan: Work together with the person to develop a safety plan. This plan should include coping strategies, emergency contacts, and steps to take during a crisis.

Identify triggers and warning signs: Help the person identify their triggers and warning signs for suicidal thoughts or behaviors. This awareness can assist in early intervention and prevention.

Remove access to lethal means: If possible, collaborate with the person to remove access to any potential lethal means, such as firearms, medications, or sharp objects.

Encourage healthy coping mechanisms: Explore and encourage healthy coping mechanisms, such as exercise, journaling, mindfulness, or engaging in activities that bring joy and relaxation.

Create a support network: Help the person build a support network of trusted individuals who can provide emotional support and intervene if needed. This network can include friends, family, or mental health professionals.

<u>Connecting with crisis hotlines and helplines</u>

Crisis hotlines and helplines are invaluable resources for immediate support during times of crisis. Here's how you can connect with these services:

Research local crisis hotlines: Familiarize yourself with local crisis hotlines and helplines that provide support for individuals at risk for suicide. Make a note of their contact information.

Encourage the person to reach out: Encourage the person to call a crisis hotline or helpline for immediate support. Assure them that trained professionals are available to listen and provide guidance.

Offer to make the call together: If the person is hesitant or unable to make the call themselves, offer to make the call together. This can help alleviate any anxiety or fear they may have.

Provide alternative communication options: If speaking on the phone is not comfortable for the person, suggest alternative communication options such as text-based crisis hotlines or online chat services.

Follow up and offer ongoing support: After connecting with a crisis hotline or helpline, follow up with the person to ensure they received the support they needed. Offer ongoing support and encourage them to continue seeking help if necessary.

Remember, providing immediate support requires a compassionate and proactive approach. By responding to crisis situations calmly, creating a supportive environment, and connecting with crisis hotlines and helplines, we can offer crucial support to individuals at risk for suicide and help guide them towards the help they need.

Mental Health and Self-Care

Taking care of our mental health is essential for overall well-being and quality of life. Here are some key practices to promote mental well-being and prioritize self-care:

Prioritize self-care: Make self-care a priority in your daily routine. This can include activities that bring you joy, relaxation, and rejuvenation, such as practicing mindfulness, engaging in hobbies, or spending time in nature.

Maintain a balanced lifestyle: Strive for a balanced lifestyle that includes healthy habits like regular exercise, nutritious eating, and sufficient sleep. These factors can positively impact your mental health.

Practice gratitude: Cultivate a gratitude practice by regularly acknowledging and appreciating the positive aspects of your life. This can help shift your focus towards the good and promote a more positive mindset.

Set boundaries: Establish healthy boundaries in your personal and professional life. Learn to say no when necessary and prioritize activities that align with your values and well-being.

Connect with others: Nurture meaningful relationships and social connections. Engage in activities that allow you to connect with others, such as joining clubs, volunteering, or participating in support groups.

Stress management techniques and coping strategies

Stress is a common part of life, but it's important to have effective strategies to manage and cope with it. Here are some techniques to help you manage stress and build resilience:

Practice relaxation techniques: Explore relaxation techniques such as deep breathing exercises, meditation, or progressive muscle relaxation. These techniques can help calm your mind and body during times of stress.

Engage in physical activity: Regular physical activity has numerous benefits for mental health. Engage in activities you enjoy, such as walking, dancing, or yoga, to reduce stress and boost your mood.

Prioritize time for hobbies: Engaging in activities you enjoy can provide a sense of fulfillment and help you unwind. Dedicate time to hobbies or creative outlets that bring you joy and allow you to express yourself.

Manage time effectively: Develop good time management skills to reduce stress and increase productivity. Prioritize tasks, break them into smaller, manageable steps, and delegate when necessary.

Seek support: Reach out to trusted friends, family, or mental health professionals for support. Talking about your feelings and concerns can provide relief and help you gain new perspectives.

<u>Encouraging help-seeking for mental health concerns</u>

Seeking help for mental health concerns is a sign of strength and an important step towards healing and well-being. Here's how you can encourage help-seeking:

Normalize the conversation: Promote open conversations about mental health to reduce stigma. Share your own experiences or stories of others who have sought help and benefited from it.

Educate about available resources: Provide information about mental health resources such as therapists, counselors, or support groups. Highlight the benefits of professional help and the variety of options available.

Offer support and empathy: Be a supportive listener and offer empathy to those who may be struggling. Let them know that you are there for them and that seeking help is a courageous step towards better mental health.

Share success stories: Share stories of individuals who have sought help and experienced positive outcomes. Hearing about others' journeys can inspire hope and encourage others to seek help.

Encourage self-reflection: Encourage individuals to reflect on their own mental well-being and recognize when they may need additional support. Encourage them to trust their instincts and seek help when they feel it is necessary.

Building Resilience and Protective Factors

Building resilience is crucial for navigating life's challenges and bouncing back from adversity. Here are some key strategies for strengthening protective factors in individuals and communities:

Promote self-awareness: Encourage individuals to develop self-awareness and recognize their strengths and abilities. This self-awareness can serve as a foundation for building resilience and facing challenges head-on.

Develop problem-solving skills: Help individuals develop effective problem-solving skills to navigate difficult situations. Encourage them to break problems into smaller, manageable steps and explore different solutions.

Encourage optimism and positive thinking: Foster a positive mindset by encouraging individuals to focus on their strengths and the potential for growth. Optimism can help individuals approach challenges with resilience and perseverance.

Provide opportunities for growth: Create opportunities for

personal growth and skill development. This can include workshops, training programs, or educational resources that empower individuals to enhance their abilities and build resilience.

Advocate for supportive environments: Advocate for supportive environments that promote resilience and well-being. This can involve policies and practices that prioritize mental health, access to resources, and social support networks.

Fostering social support networks and healthy relationships

Social support networks and healthy relationships play a vital role in building resilience. Here are some ways to foster social support and cultivate healthy relationships:

Encourage open communication: Promote open and honest communication within relationships. Encourage individuals to express their needs, concerns, and emotions, and actively listen to others without judgment.

Build a support network: Encourage individuals to build a diverse support network of trusted friends, family, and mentors. These relationships can provide emotional support, guidance, and a sense of belonging.

Participate in community activities: Engage in community activities and events that foster connections and social interactions. This can include volunteering, joining clubs or organizations, or attending local gatherings.

Practice active empathy: Encourage individuals to practice empathy and understanding towards others. This can strengthen relationships and create a supportive environment where individuals feel heard and valued.

Seek professional help when needed: Encourage individuals to seek professional help when facing challenges that may require additional support. Mental health professionals can provide guidance and help individuals develop coping strategies.

<u>Promoting positive coping skills and healthy habits</u>

Promoting positive coping skills and healthy habits is essential for building resilience. Here are some strategies to promote healthy coping skills and habits:

Encourage self-care practices: Emphasize the importance of self-care and encourage individuals to prioritize activities that promote relaxation, stress reduction, and overall well-being. This can include activities like exercise, meditation, or engaging in hobbies.

Teach stress management techniques: Educate individuals on stress management techniques such as deep breathing exercises, mindfulness, or journaling. These techniques can help individuals cope with stress and build resilience.

Promote healthy lifestyle choices: Encourage individuals to make healthy lifestyle choices, including nutritious eating, regular physical activity, and sufficient sleep. These habits can positively impact mental and physical well-being.

Provide resources for coping strategies: Share resources and information on healthy coping strategies, such as problem-solving techniques, cognitive reframing, or seeking social support. These tools can empower individuals to navigate challenges effectively.

Model healthy behaviors: Lead by example and model healthy coping skills and habits. When individuals see positive behaviors in action, they are more likely to adopt them themselves.

Reducing Stigma and Promoting Awareness

Reducing stigma surrounding suicide and mental health is crucial for creating a supportive and understanding society. Here are some ways we can challenge societal stigma:

Promote open conversations: Encourage open and non-judgmental conversations about suicide and mental health. By creating a safe space for discussion, we can help break down the barriers of stigma and encourage empathy and understanding.

Share personal stories: Share personal stories of individuals who have experienced mental health challenges or have been affected by suicide. These stories humanize the issue and help others realize that mental health struggles can affect anyone.

Educate about mental health: Provide accurate information about mental health conditions, their causes, and available treatments. By increasing awareness and understanding, we can combat misconceptions and challenge stigmatizing beliefs.

Challenge stereotypes: Challenge stereotypes and misconceptions about mental health. Encourage others to see individuals with mental health conditions as whole people, not defined solely by their diagnosis.

Support mental health campaigns: Participate in and support mental health campaigns and initiatives that aim to reduce stigma. By joining forces with organizations and individuals advocating for change, we can amplify our impact.

<u>Educating others about suicide prevention</u>

Education plays a vital role in suicide prevention. By increasing awareness and knowledge, we can empower individuals to recognize warning signs and take action. Here are some ways to educate others about suicide prevention:

Provide resources: Share reliable resources on suicide prevention, such as hotlines, websites, and educational materials. Make these resources easily accessible to those who may need them.

Offer training programs: Encourage individuals to participate in suicide prevention training programs, such as Mental Health First Aid or QPR (Question, Persuade, Refer). These programs provide valuable skills and knowledge to identify and support someone in crisis.

Organize workshops and seminars: Organize workshops and seminars on suicide prevention in schools, workplaces, and community centers. These events can provide a platform for education, discussion, and the sharing of personal experiences.

Engage in awareness campaigns: Participate in suicide prevention awareness campaigns, such as World Suicide Prevention Day or Mental Health Awareness Month. Use social media platforms to share information, resources, and personal stories.

Encourage help-seeking: Emphasize the importance of seeking help and provide information on how to access mental health services. Encourage individuals to reach out to professionals or trusted support networks when they or someone they know is in distress.

<u>Advocating for policy changes and community initiatives</u>

Advocacy for policy changes and community initiatives is essential for creating a supportive environment for mental health and suicide prevention. Here are some ways to advocate for change:

Stay informed: Stay up-to-date with mental health policies and legislation in your community. Educate yourself on current initiatives and advocate for changes that prioritize mental health and suicide prevention.

Join advocacy organizations: Join local or national advocacy organizations focused on mental health and suicide prevention. These organizations provide opportunities to collaborate with like-minded individuals and have a greater impact through collective efforts.

Write to policymakers: Write letters or emails to policymakers expressing your concerns and advocating for improved mental health policies. Share personal stories and provide evidence-based arguments to support your cause.

Participate in community initiatives: Get involved in community initiatives that promote mental health awareness and suicide prevention. This can include volunteering for helplines, participating in fundraising events, or supporting local mental health organizations.

Engage with the media: Engage with the media to raise awareness about mental health and suicide prevention. Write op-eds, share personal stories, or participate in interviews to help shape public discourse and challenge stigma.

Supporting Survivors

Supporting suicide survivors requires a compassionate and understanding approach. Here are some key points to consider when addressing the unique needs of suicide survivors:

Acknowledge the complexity of grief: Understand that grief experienced by suicide survivors can be complex and overwhelming. It may involve feelings of guilt, confusion, anger, and a sense of profound loss. Recognize that each individual's grief journey is unique and may require different forms of support.

Avoid judgment and blame: Create a safe and non-judgmental space for survivors to express their emotions and share their experiences. Avoid making assumptions or placing blame, as this can further exacerbate their pain. Instead, offer empathy, compassion, and a listening ear.

Educate yourself about suicide bereavement: Educate yourself about suicide bereavement to better understand the specific challenges faced by survivors. This knowledge will help you provide appropriate support and resources.

Respect cultural and religious differences: Be mindful of

cultural and religious differences when supporting suicide survivors. Recognize that rituals, beliefs, and coping mechanisms may vary, and respect their individual preferences.

Providing support and resources for grieving individuals

Supporting grieving individuals requires a comprehensive approach that addresses their emotional, practical, and informational needs. Here are some ways to provide support and resources for grieving suicide survivors:

Offer a listening ear: Be present and actively listen to survivors as they share their thoughts and emotions. Let them know that their feelings are valid and that you are there to support them.

Connect survivors with support groups: Connect survivors with support groups specifically designed for those who have lost a loved one to suicide. These groups provide a safe space for individuals to share their experiences, receive validation, and find comfort in the company of others who have gone through similar losses.

Provide access to counseling services: Offer information and resources for professional counseling services specializing in grief and trauma. Therapy can provide survivors with a safe and confidential space to process their emotions and develop coping strategies.

Share educational materials: Provide survivors with educational materials on grief and suicide bereavement. These resources can help them understand their own emotions and navigate the grieving process.

Offer practical assistance: Offer practical assistance to survivors, such as helping with funeral arrangements, organizing meals, or providing transportation. These acts of kindness can alleviate some of the burdens they may be facing during this difficult time.

<u>Nurturing healing and resilience in survivors</u>

Nurturing healing and resilience in suicide survivors is essential for their long-term well-being. Here are some strategies to promote healing and resilience:

Encourage self-care: Emphasize the importance of self-care and encourage survivors to engage in activities that promote their physical, emotional, and mental well-being. This can include exercise, relaxation techniques, journaling, or engaging in hobbies.

Promote healthy coping mechanisms: Help survivors develop healthy coping mechanisms to navigate their grief. This can include encouraging them to express their emotions through creative outlets, such as art or writing, or engaging in activities that bring them joy and a sense of purpose.

Facilitate connections with others: Encourage survivors to connect with others who have experienced similar losses. This can be through support groups, online communities, or peer mentoring programs. Building connections with others who understand their pain can provide a sense of validation and support.

Provide information on self-help resources: Share information on self-help resources, such as books, podcasts, or online courses, that focus on grief and resilience. These resources can empower survivors to continue their healing journey and develop their own strategies for resilience.

Promote professional help when needed: Encourage survivors to seek professional help if they are struggling with their mental health or finding it challenging to cope with their grief. Mental health professionals can provide specialized support and guidance tailored to their individual needs.

Prevention Strategies and Community Involvement

Preventing suicide requires a multi-faceted approach that combines evidence-based strategies to address risk factors and promote protective factors. Here are some key prevention strategies to consider:

Promote mental health awareness: Increase awareness about mental health and the importance of seeking help. Encourage open conversations about mental health in schools, workplaces, and communities to reduce stigma and encourage early intervention.

Identify and support at-risk individuals: Train individuals to recognize warning signs of suicide and provide them with the skills to intervene appropriately. This can include gatekeeper training programs like QPR (Question, Persuade, Refer) or Mental Health First Aid.

Enhance access to mental health services: Improve access to mental health services by reducing barriers such as cost, stigma, and limited availability. Advocate for increased funding and resources for mental health programs and services.

Restrict access to lethal means: Implement measures to restrict access to lethal means of self-harm, such as firearms or medications. This can include safe storage practices, education on responsible medication use, and implementing policies to reduce access to lethal means.

School-based interventions and community education programs

Schools and community education programs play a vital role in suicide prevention. By equipping individuals with knowledge and skills, we can create a supportive environment that promotes mental health and well-being. Here are some effective interventions:

Implement mental health curriculum in schools: Integrate mental health education into school curricula, teaching students about mental health, coping strategies, and how to seek help. This helps reduce stigma and equips students with the knowledge to support themselves and their peers.

Train teachers and staff: Provide training to teachers and school staff on recognizing signs of distress, responding to students in crisis, and connecting them to appropriate resources. This training ensures that schools are equipped to support students' mental health needs.

Establish peer support programs: Implement peer support programs where students can receive support from trained peers. These programs create a safe and confidential space for students to share their struggles and seek guidance from their peers.

Engage parents and caregivers: Educate parents and caregivers about suicide prevention and mental health. Offer workshops and resources to help them recognize warning signs and provide support to their children. Parental involvement is crucial in creating a supportive network for students.

<u>Getting involved in local suicide prevention efforts</u>

Community involvement is essential for effective suicide prevention. By coming together and taking action, we can make a significant impact on the well-being of our communities. Here are some ways to get involved:

Join local suicide prevention organizations: Connect with local suicide prevention organizations and volunteer your time and skills. These organizations often organize events, awareness campaigns, and support services for individuals in need.

Participate in fundraising events: Support local suicide prevention efforts by participating in fundraising events. This can include walks, runs, or other community activities that raise funds and awareness for suicide prevention programs.

Advocate for policy changes: Get involved in advocacy efforts to promote mental health policies and legislation. Write letters to policymakers, attend community meetings, and share your personal experiences to advocate for change.

Organize community education programs: Take the initiative to organize community education programs on suicide prevention. This can include workshops, seminars, or panel discussions where experts and community members come together to share knowledge and resources.

Promote helpline services: Spread awareness about helpline services available in your community. Share information about crisis hotlines, text lines, and online chat services that provide immediate support to individuals in crisis.

Inspiring Stories of Hope and Recovery

As a therapist, I have had the privilege of witnessing incredible stories of hope and recovery from individuals who have faced the depths of despair and emerged stronger than ever. These stories serve as a testament to the resilience of the human spirit and the power of support and treatment. Here are a few inspiring stories that have touched my heart:

Sarah's Journey of Healing: Sarah came to me feeling utterly defeated by her battle with depression. She had attempted suicide multiple times and believed that her life was devoid of purpose. Through therapy, Sarah gradually began to uncover the underlying issues contributing to her depression. With time, patience, and a strong support system, she learned coping strategies, developed a renewed sense of self-worth, and discovered her passion for helping others. Today, Sarah is a mental health advocate, sharing her story to inspire hope in others who may be struggling.

Mark's Triumph Over Addiction: Mark's life had spiraled out of control due to his addiction to drugs and alcohol. He had hit rock bottom and contemplated suicide as a way out. With the support of his family and a dedicated treatment team,

Mark embarked on a journey of recovery. Through therapy, he learned to confront his underlying emotional pain and develop healthier coping mechanisms. Today, Mark is a living testament to the power of perseverance and is actively involved in supporting others on their own paths to recovery.

Emily's Transformation Through Connection: Emily had battled with feelings of isolation and despair for years. She believed that she was a burden to those around her and contemplated ending her life. Through therapy, Emily gradually built a strong therapeutic relationship, which provided her with a safe space to share her deepest fears and insecurities. With time, she began to develop meaningful connections with others who had experienced similar struggles. These connections became a lifeline for Emily, reminding her that she was not alone. Today, Emily is an advocate for mental health awareness, using her story to inspire others to seek help and find connection.

These stories highlight the transformative power of therapy, support, and personal resilience. They remind us that even in the darkest moments, there is hope for a brighter future. Each individual's journey is unique, but they all share a common thread of strength and the willingness to seek help. As a therapist, I am humbled by the privilege of being a part of these stories and witnessing the incredible transformations that can occur when hope is nurtured and recovery is embraced.

Conclusion

Throughout this book, we have explored the critical topic of recognizing the warning signs of suicide. By understanding the common warning signs, behavioral cues, and the role of risk and protective factors, we can play an active role in suicide prevention and support those in need.

Let's recap the key points we have discussed:

We have identified common warning signs of suicide, such as changes in behavior, extreme mood swings, and talking about death or suicide.

We have highlighted behavioral, emotional, and verbal cues to watch for, including expressing feelings of hopelessness, withdrawing from loved ones, and engaging in risky behaviors.

We have recognized the role of risk factors, such as mental health disorders and previous suicide attempts, as well as protective factors like strong social support and access to mental health care.

It is crucial to remember that suicide prevention is a collective effort. Each and every one of us has the power to make a difference.

Now, I encourage you to take action. Here are some ways you can contribute to suicide prevention:

Educate yourself: Continue to learn about suicide prevention, warning signs, and available resources. The more knowledge you have, the better equipped you will be to support those in need.

Be observant: Pay attention to the people around you. Take notice of any changes in their behavior, mood, or demeanor. Trust your instincts and don't hesitate to reach out if you suspect someone may be struggling.

Listen with empathy: Create a safe and non-judgmental space for others to share their thoughts and feelings. Sometimes, simply lending an empathetic ear can make a world of difference.

Offer support: Let those who are struggling know that they are not alone. Offer your support, whether it's through a kind word, a helping hand, or connecting them with professional resources.

Advocate for mental health: Raise awareness about mental health and the importance of seeking help. Challenge the stigma surrounding mental health issues and promote a culture of understanding and acceptance.

Remember, even the smallest acts of kindness and support can have a profound impact on someone's life. By taking action, we can create a world where individuals in distress feel seen, heard, and supported.

Recognizing the warning signs of suicide is a crucial step in suicide prevention. By staying vigilant, offering support, and advocating for mental health, we can make a difference and save lives. Together, let's create a future where hope triumphs over despair and where every individual knows they are not alone in their struggles.

Thanks

Dear Reader,

Thank you for taking the time to read this book on recognizing the warning signs of suicide. I hope that the information provided has been valuable and insightful for you.

If you found this book helpful and informative, I kindly ask you to consider leaving a review or sharing your thoughts. Your feedback is incredibly valuable and can help others discover this resource as well. By sharing your positive experience, you can play a part in spreading awareness about suicide prevention and supporting those in need.

Furthermore, I encourage you to share this book with your friends, family, and colleagues. By passing along this knowl-edge, you can contribute to a wider understanding of suicide prevention and potentially make a difference in someone's life.

Remember, together we can create a world where compassion, understanding, and support are readily available to those who need it most. Thank you once again for your time and dedication to this important topic.

With gratitude,

Dr. Stephanie D. Ward